Ketogenic Side Dish

Recipes

***Effective Low-Carb Recipes To
Balance Hormones And Effortlessly
Reach Your Weight Loss Goal.***

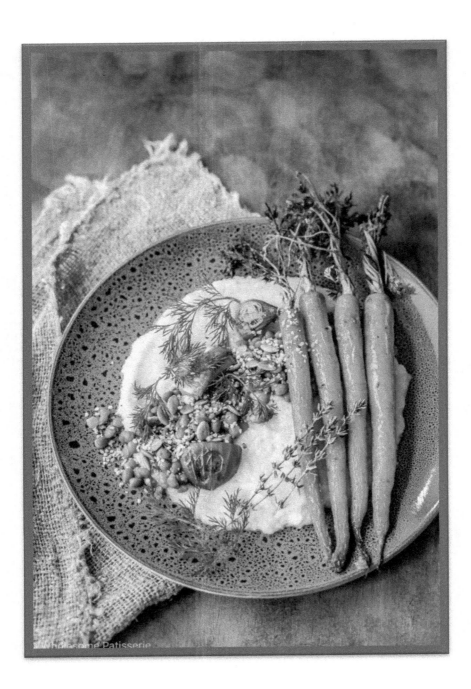

Introduction

Do you want to make a change in your life? Do you want to become a healthier person who can enjoy a new and improved life? Then, you are definitely in the right place. You are about to discover a wonderful and very healthy diet that has changed millions of lives. We are talking about the Ketogenic diet, a lifestyle that will mesmerize you and that will make you a new person in no time.

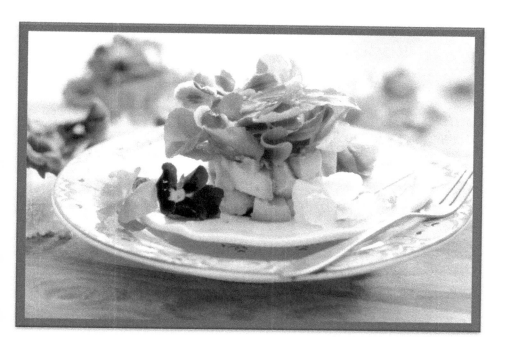

So, let's sit back, relax and find out more about the Ketogenic diet.

A keto diet is a low carb one. This is the first and one of the most important things you should now. During such a diet, your body makes ketones in your liver and these are used as energy.

Your body will produce less insulin and glucose and a state of ketosis is induced. Ketosis is a natural process that appears when our food intake is lower than usual. The body will soon adapt to this state and therefore you will be able to lose weight in no time but you will also become healthier and your physical and mental performances will improve.

Your blood sugar levels will improve and you won't be predisposed to diabetes. Also, epilepsy and heart diseases can be prevented if you are on a Ketogenic diet.

Your cholesterol will improve and you will feel amazing in no time.

How does that sound

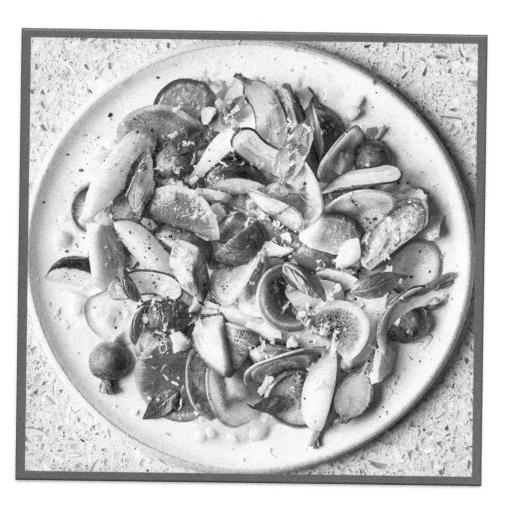

A Ketogenic diet is simple and easy to follow as long as you follow some simple rules. You don't need to make huge changes but there are some things you should know.

So, here goes!

Now let's start our magical culinary journey!

Ketogenic lifestyle...here we come!

Enjoy!

Simple Kimchi

Serve this with a steak!

Preparation time: 1 hour and 10 minutes **Cooking time:** 0 minutes **Servings:** 6

Ingredients:

- 3 tablespoons salt
- 1 pound napa cabbage, chopped
- 1 carrot, julienned
- ½ cup daikon radish
- 3 green onion stalks, chopped
- 1 tablespoon fish sauce
- 3 tablespoons chili flakes
- 3 garlic cloves, minced
- 1 tablespoon sesame oil
- ½ inch ginger, grated

Directions:

1. In a bowl, mix cabbage with the salt, massage well for 10 minutes, cover and leave aside for 1 hour.
2. In a bowl, mix chili flakes with fish sauce, garlic, sesame oil and ginger and stir very well.
3. Drain cabbage well, rinses under cold water and transfer to a bowl.
4. Add carrots, green onions, radish and chili paste and stir everything.
5. Leave in a dark and cold place for at least 2 days before serving as a side for a keto steak.

Enjoy!

Nutrition: calories 60, fat 3, fiber 2, carbs 5, protein 1

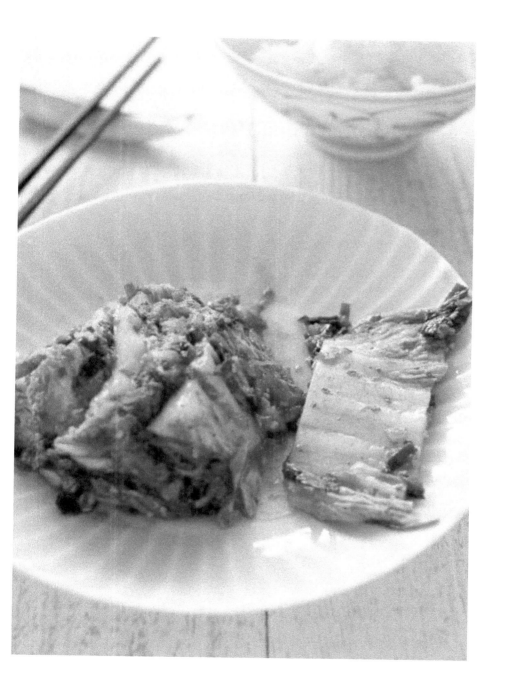

Delicious Green Beans Side Dish

You will definitely enjoy this great side dish!

Preparation time: 10 minutes **Cooking time:** 10 minutes **Servings:** 4

Ingredients:

- 2/3 cup parmesan, grated
- 1 egg
- 12 ounces green beans
- Salt and black pepper to the taste
- ½ teaspoon garlic powder
- ¼ teaspoon paprika

Directions:

1. In a bowl, mix parmesan with salt, pepper, garlic powder and paprika and stir.
2. In another bowl, whisk the egg with salt and pepper.
3. Dredge green beans in egg and then in parmesan mix.
4. Place green beans on a lined baking sheet, introduce in the oven at 400 degrees F for 10 minutes.
5. Serve hot as a side dish.

Enjoy!

Nutrition: calories 114, fat 5, fiber 7, carbs 3, protein 9

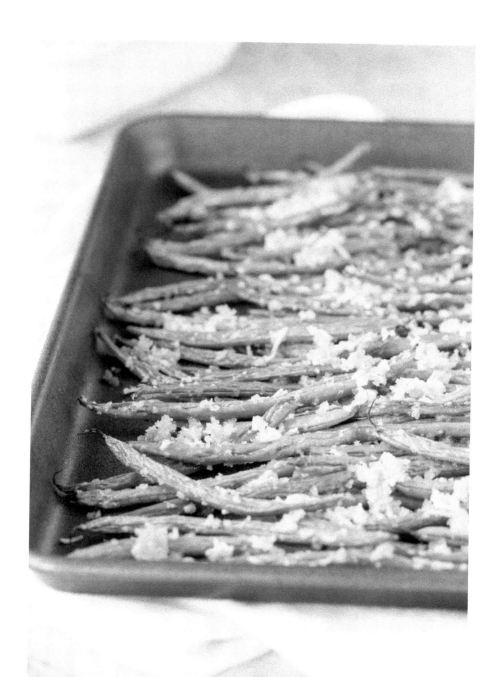

Simple Cauliflower Mash

This simple Ketogenic mash goes with a meat based dish!

Preparation time: 10 minutes **Cooking time:** 10 minutes **Servings:** 2

Ingredients:
- ¼ cup sour cream
- 1 small cauliflower head, florets separated
- Salt and black pepper to the taste
- 2 tablespoons feta cheese, crumbled
- 2 tablespoons black olives, pitted and sliced

Directions:

1. Put water in a pot, add some salt, bring to a boil over medium heat, add florets, cook for 10 minutes, take off heat and drain.
2. Return cauliflower to the pot, add salt and black pepper to the taste and the sour cream and blend suing an immersion blender.
3. Add black olives and feta cheese, stir and serve as a side dish.

Enjoy!

Nutrition: calories 100, fat 4, fiber 2, carbs 3, protein 2

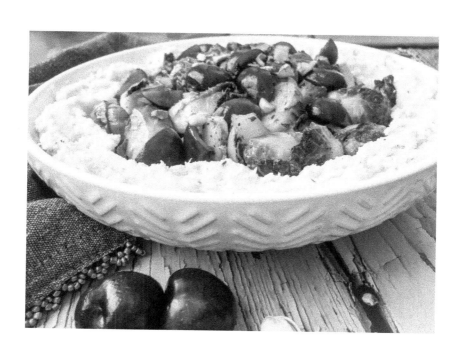

Delicious Portobello Mushrooms

These are simply the best! It's a great keto side dish!

Preparation time: 10 minutes **Cooking time:** 10 minutes **Servings:** 4

Ingredients:
- 12 ounces Portobello mushrooms, sliced
- Salt and black pepper to the taste
- ½ teaspoon basil, dried
- 2 tablespoons olive oil
- ½ teaspoon tarragon, dried
- ½ teaspoon rosemary, dried
- ½ teaspoon thyme, dried
- 2 tablespoons balsamic vinegar

Directions:
1. In a bowl, mix oil with vinegar, salt, pepper, rosemary, tarragon, basil and thyme and whisk well.
2. Add mushroom slices, toss to coat well, place them on your preheated grill over medium high heat, cook for 5 minutes on both sides and serve as a keto side dish.

Enjoy!

Nutrition: calories 80, fat 4, fiber 4, carbs 2, protein 4

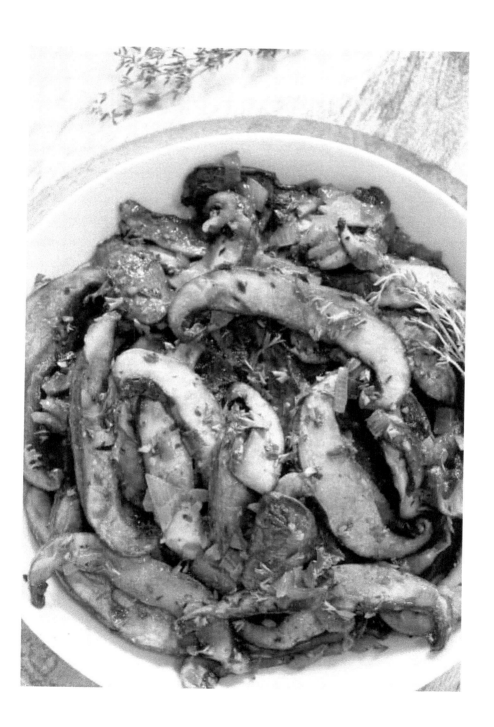

Brussels Sprouts Side Dish

This is an Asian-style side dish you must try!

Preparation time: 10 minutes **Cooking time:** 10 minutes **Servings:** 4

Ingredients:

- 1 pound Brussels sprouts, trimmed and halved
- Salt and black pepper to the taste
- 1 teaspoon sesame seeds
- 1 tablespoon green onions, chopped
- 1 and ½ tablespoons sukrin gold syrup
- 1 tablespoon coconut aminos
- 2 tablespoons sesame oil
- 1 tablespoon sriracha

Directions:

1. In a bowl, mix sesame oil with coconut aminos, sriracha, syrup, salt and black pepper and whisk well.
2. Heat up a pan over medium high heat, add Brussels sprouts and cook them for 5 minutes on each side.
3. Add sesame oil mix, toss to coat, sprinkle sesame seeds and green onions, stir again and serve as a side dish.

Enjoy!

Nutrition: calories 110, fat 4, fiber 4, carbs 6, protein 4

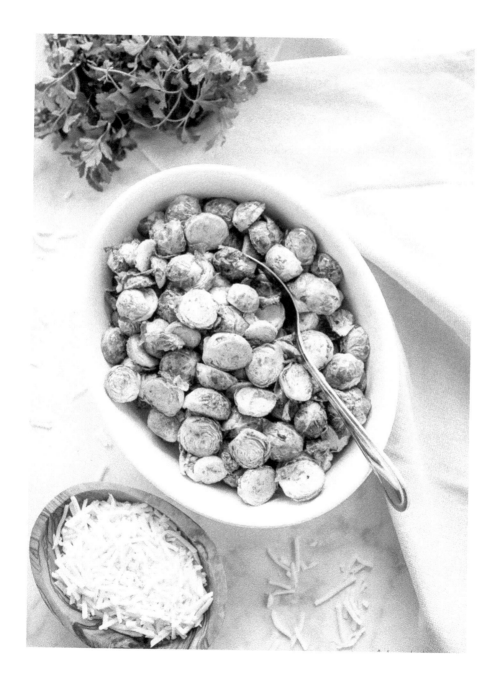

Delicious Pesto

This keto pesto can be served with a tasty chicken dish!

Preparation time: 10 minutes **Cooking time:** 0 minutes **Servings:** 4

Ingredients:
- ½ cup olive oil
- 2 cups basil
- 1/3 cup pine nuts
- 1/3 cup parmesan cheese, grated
- 2 garlic cloves, chopped
- Salt and black pepper to the taste

Directions:
1. Put basil in your food processor, add pine nuts and garlic and blend very well.
2. Add parmesan, salt, pepper and the oil gradually and blend again until you obtain a paste.
3. Serve with chicken!

Enjoy!

Nutrition: calories 100, fat 7, fiber 3, carbs 1, protein 5

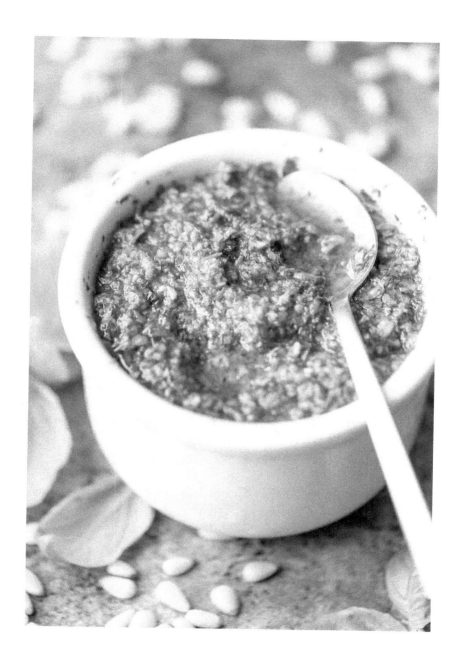

Brussels Sprouts And Bacon

You will love Brussels sprouts from now on!

Preparation time: 10 minutes **Cooking time:** 30 minutes **Servings:** 4

Ingredients:
- 8 bacon strips, chopped
- 1 pound Brussels sprouts, trimmed and halved
- Salt and black pepper to the taste
- A pinch of cumin, ground
- A pinch of red pepper, crushed
- 2 tablespoons extra virgin olive oil

Directions:
1. In a bowl, mix Brussels sprouts with salt, pepper, cumin, red pepper and oil and toss to coat.
2. Spread Brussels sprouts on a lined baking sheet, introduce in the oven at 375 degrees F and bake for 30 minutes.
3. Meanwhile, heat up a pan over medium heat, add bacon pieces and cook them until they become crispy.
4. Divide baked Brussels sprouts on plates, top with bacon and serve as a side dish right away.

Enjoy!

Nutrition: calories 256, fat 20, fiber 6, carbs 5, protein 15

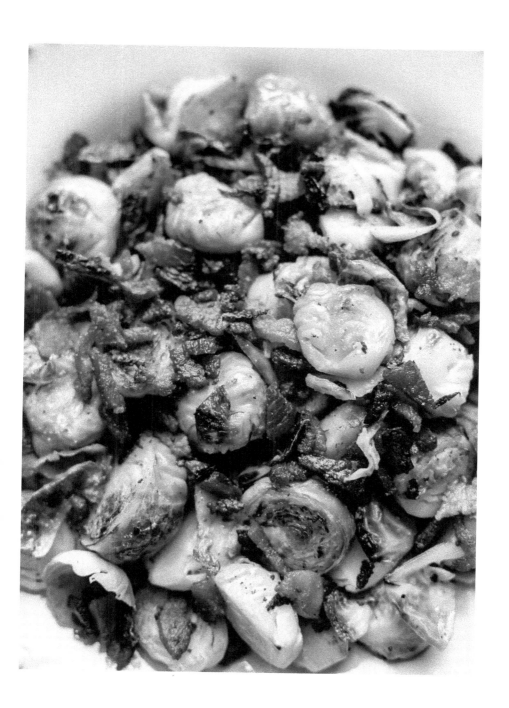

Delicious Spinach Side Dish

This is very creamy and tasty!

Preparation time: 10 minutes **Cooking time:** 15 minutes **Servings:** 2

Ingredients:
- 2 garlic cloves, minced
- 8 ounces spinach leaves
- A drizzle of olive oil
- Salt and black pepper to the taste
- 4 tablespoons sour cream
- 1 tablespoon ghee
- 2 tablespoons parmesan cheese, grated

Directions:

1. Heat up a pan with the oil over medium heat, add spinach, stir and cook until it softens.
2. Add salt, pepper, ghee, parmesan and ghee, stir and cook for 4 minutes.
3. Add sour cream, stir and cook for 5 minutes more.
4. Divide between plates and serve as a side dish.

Enjoy!

Nutrition: calories 133, fat 10, fiber 4, carbs 4, protein 2

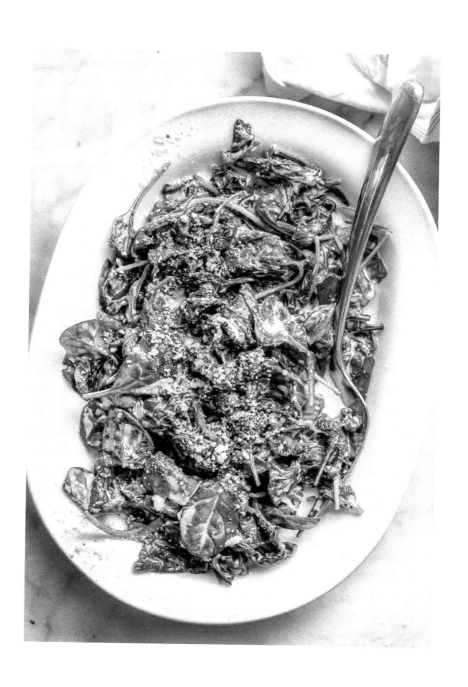

Amazing Avocado Fries

Try them as a side dish for a delicious steak!

Preparation time: 10 minutes **Cooking time:** 5 minutes **Servings:** 3

Ingredients:
- 3 avocados, pitted, peeled, halved and sliced
- 1 and ½ cups sunflower oil
- 1 and ½ cups almond meal
- A pinch of cayenne pepper
- Salt and black pepper to the taste

Directions:
1. In a bowl mix almond meal with salt, pepper and cayenne and stir.
2. In a second bowl, whisk eggs with a pinch of salt and pepper.
3. Dredge avocado pieces in egg and then in almond meal mix.
4. Heat up a pan with the oil over medium high heat, add avocado fries and cook them until they are golden.
5. Transfer to paper towels, drain grease and divide between plates.
6. Serve as a side dish.

Enjoy!

Nutrition: calories 450, fat 43, fiber 4, carbs 7, protein 17

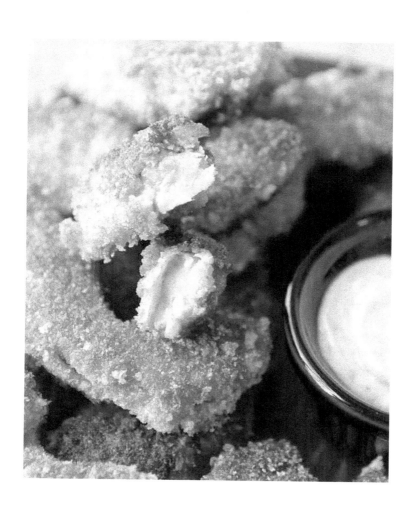

Simple Roasted Cauliflower

This is so delicious and very easy to make at home! It's a great keto side dish!

Preparation time: 10 minutes **Cooking time:** 25 minutes **Servings:** 6

Ingredients:

- 1 cauliflower head, florets separated
- Salt and black pepper to the taste
- 1/3 cup parmesan, grated
- 1 tablespoon parsley, chopped
- 3 tablespoons olive oil
- 2 tablespoons extra virgin olive oil

Directions:

1. In a bowl, mix oil with garlic, salt, pepper and cauliflower florets.
2. Toss to coat well, spread this on a lined baking sheet, introduce in the oven at 450 degrees F and bake for 25 minutes, stirring halfway.
3. Add parmesan and parsley, stir and cook for 5 minutes more.
4. Divide between plates and serve as a keto side dish.

Enjoy!

Nutrition: calories 118, fat 2, fiber 3, carbs 1, protein 6

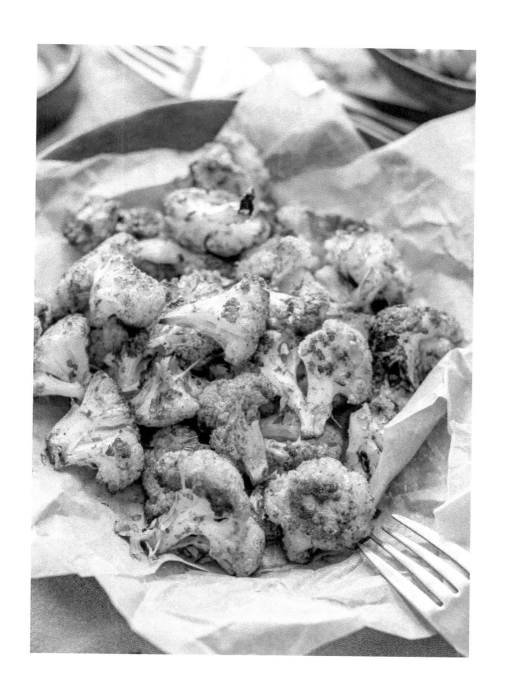

Mushroom And Spinach Side Dish

This is an Italian style keto side dish worth trying as soon as possible!

Preparation time: 10 minutes **Cooking time:** 10 minutes **Servings:** 4

Ingredients:
- 10 ounces spinach leaves, chopped
- Salt and black pepper to the taste
- 14 ounces mushrooms, chopped
- 2 garlic cloves, minced
- A handful parsley, chopped
- 1 yellow onion, chopped
- 4 tablespoons olive oil
- 2 tablespoons balsamic vinegar

Directions:
1. Heat up a pan with the oil over medium high heat, add garlic and onion, stir and cook for 4 minutes.
2. Add mushrooms, stir and cook for 3 minutes more.
3. Add spinach, stir and cook for 3 minutes.
4. Add vinegar, salt and pepper, stir and cook for 1 minute more.
5. Add parsley, stir, divide between plates and serve hot as a side dish.

Enjoy!

Nutrition: calories 200, fat 4, fiber 6, carbs 2, protein 12

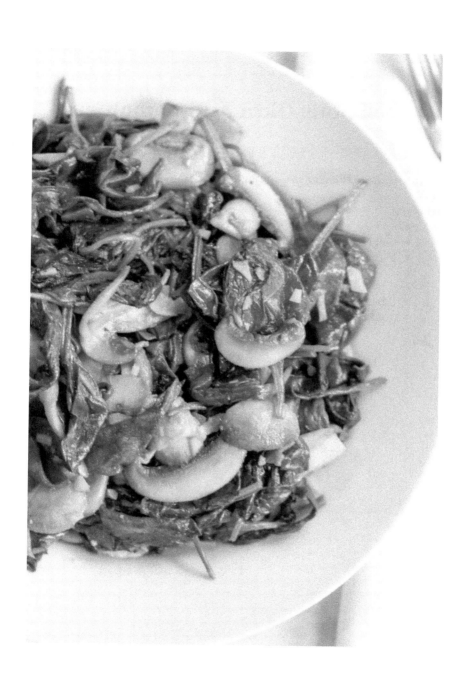

Delicious Okra And Tomatoes

This is very simple and easy to make! It's one of the best keto sides ever!

Preparation time: 10 minutes **Cooking time:** 10 minutes **Servings:** 6

Ingredients:
- 14 ounces canned stewed tomatoes, chopped
- Salt and black pepper to the taste
- 2 celery stalks, chopped
- 1 yellow onion, chopped
- 1 pound okra, sliced
- 2 bacon slices, chopped
- 1 small green bell peppers, chopped

Directions:

1. Heat up a pan over medium high heat, add bacon, stir, brown for a few minutes, transfer to paper towels and leave aside for now.
2. Heat up the pan again over medium heat, add okra, bell pepper, onion and celery, stir and cook for 2 minutes.
3. Add tomatoes, salt and pepper, stir and cook for 3 minutes.
4. Divide on plates, garnish with crispy bacon and serve.

Enjoy!

Nutrition: calories 100, fat 2, fiber 3, carbs 2, protein 6

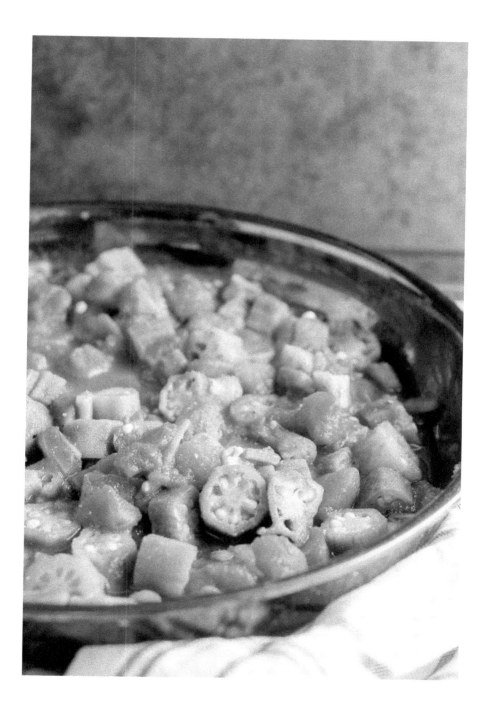

Amazing Snap Peas And Mint

This side dish is not just a keto one! It's a simple and quick one as well!

Preparation time: 10 minutes **Cooking time:** 5 minutes **Servings:** 4

Ingredients:
- ¾ pound sugar snap peas, trimmed
- Salt and black pepper to the taste
- 1 tablespoon mint leaves, chopped
- 2 teaspoons olive oil
- 3 green onions, chopped
- 1 garlic clove, minced

Directions:
1. Heat up a pan with the oil over medium high heat.
2. Add snap peas, salt, pepper, green onions, garlic and mint.
3. Stir everything, cook for 5 minutes, divide between plates and serve as a side dish for a pork steak.

Enjoy!

Nutrition: calories 70, fat 1, fiber 1, carbs 0.4, protein 6

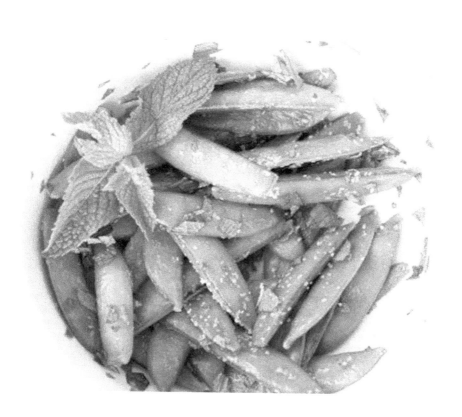

Collard Greens Side Dish

This is just unbelievably amazing!

Preparation time: 10 minutes **Cooking time:** 2 hours and 15 minutes **Servings:** 10

Ingredients:
- 5 bunches collard greens, chopped
- Salt and black pepper to the taste
- 1 tablespoon red pepper flakes, crushed
- 5 cups chicken stock
- 1 turkey leg
- 2 tablespoons garlic, minced
- ¼ cup olive oil

Directions:

1. Heat up a pot with the oil over medium heat, add garlic, stir and cook for 1 minute.
2. Add stock, salt, pepper and turkey leg, stir, cover and simmer for 30 minutes.
3. Add collard greens, cover pot again and cook for 45 minutes more.
4. Reduce heat to medium, add more salt and pepper, stir and cook for 1 hour.
5. Drain greens, mix them with red pepper flakes, stir, divide between plates and serve as a side dish.

Enjoy!

Nutrition: calories 143, fat 3, fiber 4, carbs 3, protein 6

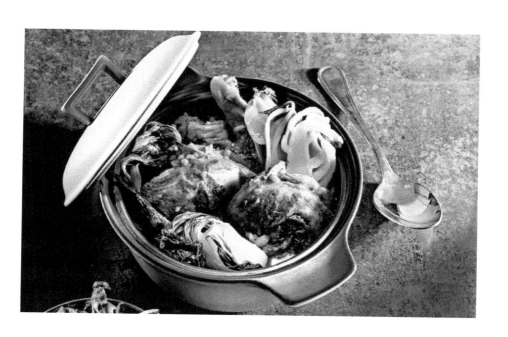

Eggplant And Tomato Side Dish

It's a keto side dish you will make over and over again!

Preparation time: 10 minutes **Cooking time:** 15 minutes **Servings:** 4

Ingredients:

- 1 tomato, sliced
- 1 eggplant, sliced into thin rounds
- Salt and black pepper to the taste
- ¼ cup parmesan, grated
- A drizzle of olive oil

Directions:

1. Place eggplant slices on a lined baking dish, drizzle some oil and sprinkle half of the parmesan.
2. Top eggplant slices with tomato ones, season with salt and pepper to the taste and sprinkle the rest of the cheese over them.
3. Introduce in the oven at 400 degrees F and bake for 15 minutes.
4. Divide between plates and serve hot as a side dish.

Enjoy!

Nutrition: calories 55, fat 1, fiber 1, carbs 0.5, protein 7

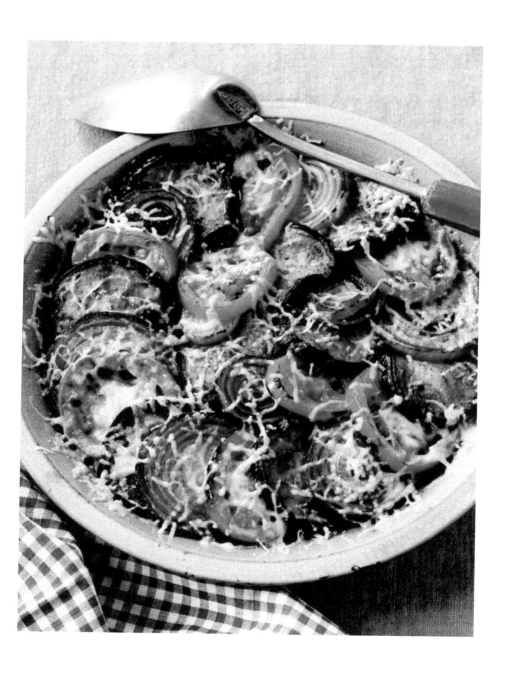

Broccoli With Lemon Almond Butter

This side dish is perfect for a grilled steak!

Preparation time: 10 minutes **Cooking time:** 10 minutes **Servings:** 4

Ingredients:
- 1 broccoli head, florets separated
- Salt and black pepper to the taste
- ¼ cup almonds, blanched
- 1 teaspoon lemon zest
- ¼ cup coconut butter, melted
- 2 tablespoons lemon juice

Directions:
1. Put water in a pot, add salt and bring to a boil over medium high heat.
2. Place broccoli florets in a steamer basket, place into the pot, cover and steam for 8 minutes.
3. Drain and transfer to a bowl.
4. Heat up a pan with the coconut butter over medium heat, add lemon juice, lemon zest and almonds, stir and take off heat.
5. Add broccoli, toss to coat, divide between plates and serve as a Ketogenic side dish.

Enjoy!

Nutrition: calories 170, fat 15, fiber 4, carbs 4, protein 4

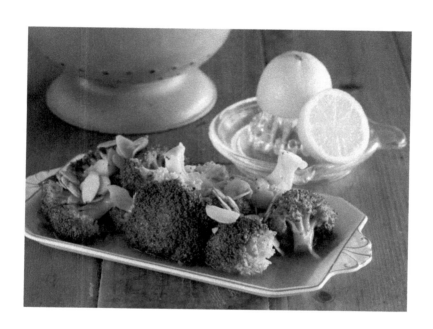

Simple Sautéed Broccoli

Serve this with some baked chicken or fish!

Preparation time: 10 minutes **Cooking time:** 22 minutes **Servings:** 4

Ingredients:
- 5 tablespoons olive oil
- 1 garlic clove, minced
- 1 pound broccoli florets
- 1 tablespoon parmesan, grated
- Salt and black pepper to the taste

Directions:
1. Put water in a pot, add salt, bring to a boil over medium high heat, add broccoli, cook for 5 minutes and drain.
2. Heat up a pan with the oil over medium high heat, add garlic, stir and cook for 2 minutes.
3. Add broccoli, stir and cook for 15 minutes.
4. Take off heat, sprinkle parmesan, divide between plates and serve.

Enjoy!

Nutrition: calories 193, fat 14, fiber 3, carbs 6, protein 5

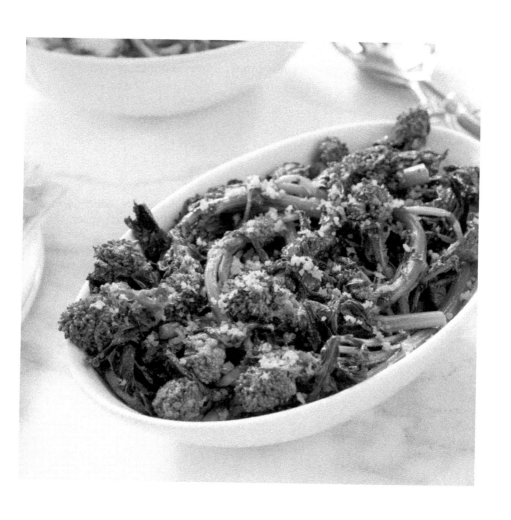

Easy Grilled Onions

This Ketogenic side dish is perfect for a steak!

Preparation time: 10 minutes **Cooking time:** 1 hour **Servings:** 4

Ingredients:
- ½ cup ghee
- 4 onions
- 4 chicken bouillon cubes
- Salt and black pepper

Direction:
1. Cut onion tops make a hole in the middle, divide ghee and chicken bouillon cubes into these holes and season with salt and pepper.
2. Wrap onions in tin foil, place them on preheated kitchen grill and grill for 1 hour.
3. Unwrap onions, chop them into big chunks, arrange on plates and serve as a side dish.

Enjoy!

Nutrition: calories 135, fat 11, fiber 4, carbs 6, protein 3

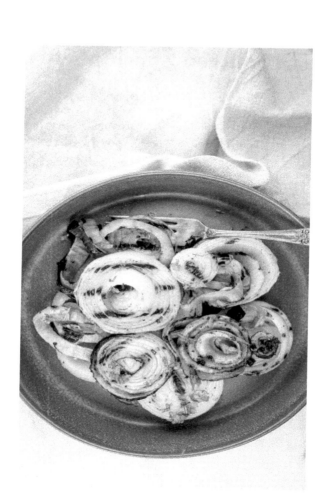

Sautéed Zucchinis

Serve them with some chicken meat and enjoy a perfect meal!

Preparation time: 10 minutes **Cooking time:** 15 minutes **Servings:** 6

Ingredients:
- 1 red onion, chopped
- 1 tomato, chopped
- ½ pound tomatoes, chopped
- Salt and black pepper to the taste
- 1 garlic clove, minced
- 1 garlic clove, minced
- 1 teaspoon Italian seasoning
- 4 zucchinis, sliced

Directions:
1. Heat up a pan with the oil over medium heat, add onion, salt and pepper, stir and cook for 2 minutes.
2. Add zucchinis, stir and cook for 5 minutes.
3. Add garlic, tomatoes and Italian seasoning, stir, cook for 6 minutes more.
4. Take off heat, divide between plates and serve as a side dish.

Enjoy!

Nutrition: calories 70, fat 3, fiber 2, carbs 6, protein 4

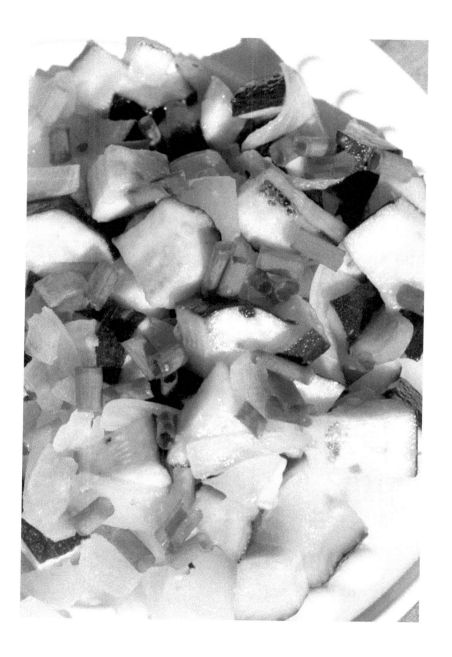

Delicious Fried Swiss Chard

You must try this keto side dish! It goes perfectly with some grilled meat!

Preparation time: 10 minutes **Cooking time:** 10 minutes **Servings:** 2

Ingredients:
- 2 tablespoons ghee
- 4 bacon slices, chopped
- 1 bunch Swiss chard, roughly chopped
- ½ teaspoon garlic paste
- 3 tablespoons lemon juice
- Salt and black pepper to the taste

Directions:
1. Heat up a pan over medium heat, add bacon pieces and cook until it's crispy.
2. Add ghee and stir until it melts.
3. Add garlic paste and lemon juice, stir and cook for 1 minute.
4. Add Swiss chard, stir and cook for 4 minutes.
5. Add salt and black pepper to the taste, stir, divide between plates and serve as a keto side dish.

Enjoy!

Nutrition: calories 300, fat 32, fiber 7, carbs 6, protein 8

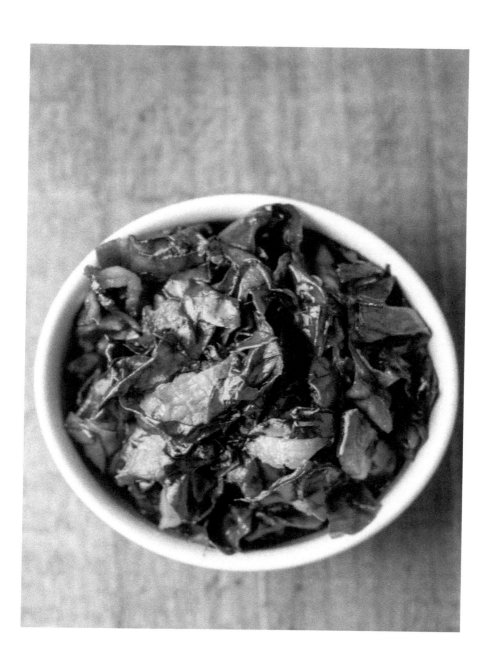

Delicious Side Mushroom Salad

This is really delicious and easy to make!

Preparation time: 10 minutes **Cooking time:** 10 minutes **Servings:** 4

Ingredients:
- 2 tablespoons ghee
- 1 pound cremini mushrooms, chopped
- 4 tablespoons extra virgin olive oil
- Salt and black pepper to the taste
- 4 bunches arugula
- 8 slices prosciutto
- 2 tablespoons apple cider vinegar
- 8 sun-dried tomatoes in oil, drained and chopped
- Some parmesan shavings
- Some parsley leaves, chopped

Directions:
1. Heat up a pan with the ghee and half of the oil over medium high heat.
2. Add mushrooms, salt and pepper, stir and cook for 3 minutes.
3. Reduce heat, stir again and cook for 3 more minutes.
4. Add the rest of the oil and the vinegar, stir and cook 1 minute more
5. Place arugula on a serving platter, add prosciutto on top, add mushroom mix, sun dried tomatoes, more salt and pepper, parmesan shavings and parsley and serve.

Enjoy!

Nutrition: calories 160, fat 4, fiber 2, carbs 2, protein 6

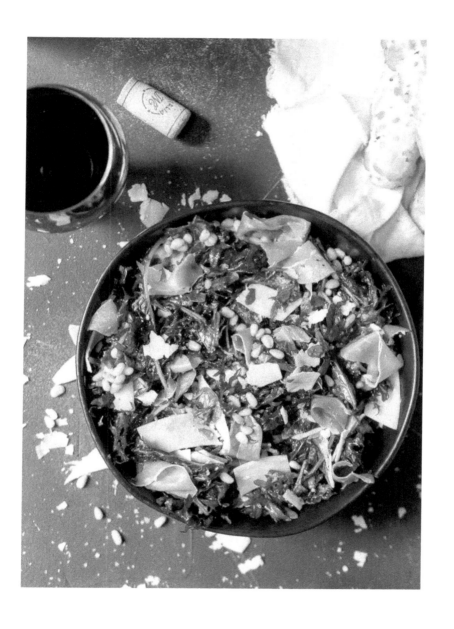

Greek Side Salad

Get ready for a fabulous combination of ingredients! Taste this amazing salad at once!

Preparation time: 10 minutes **Cooking time:** 7 minutes **Servings:** 6

Ingredients:
- ½ pounds mushrooms, sliced
- 1 tablespoon extra virgin olive oil
- 3 garlic cloves, minced
- 1 teaspoon basil, dried
- Salt and black pepper to the taste
- 1 tomato, diced
- 3 tablespoons lemon juice
- ½ cup water
- 1 tablespoons coriander, chopped

Directions:
1. Heat up a pan with the oil over medium heat, add mushrooms, stir and cook for 3 minutes.
2. Add basil and garlic, stir and cook for 1 minute more.
3. Add water, salt, pepper, tomato and lemon juice, stir and cook for a few minutes more.
4. Take off heat, transfer to a bowl, leave aside to cool down, sprinkle coriander and serve.

Enjoy!

Nutrition: calories 200, fat 2, fiber 2, carbs 1, protein 10

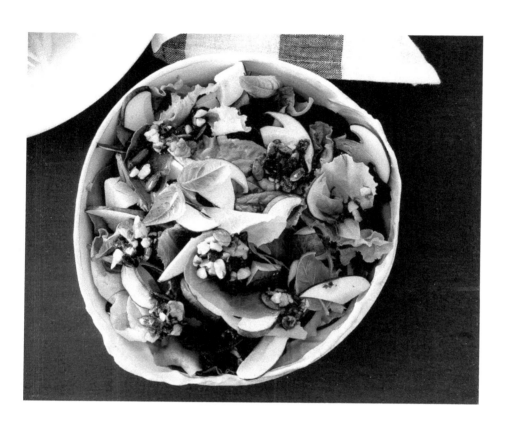

Tomato Salsa

It's a perfect and most simple keto side dish!

Preparation time: 2 hours **Cooking time:** 0 minutes **Servings:** 5

Ingredients:
- 3 yellow tomatoes, seedless and chopped
- 1 red tomato, seedless and chopped
- Salt and black pepper to the taste
- 1 cup watermelon, seedless and chopped
- 1/3 cup red onion, finely chopped
- 1 mango, peeled, seedless and chopped
- 2 jalapeno peppers, finely chopped
- ¼ cup cilantro, finely chopped
- 3 tablespoons lime juice
- 2 teaspoons honey

Directions:
1. In a bowl, mix yellow and red tomatoes with mango, watermelon, onion and jalapeno.
2. Add cilantro, lime juice, salt, pepper to the taste and honey and stir well.
3. Cover bowl, keep in the fridge for 2 hours and then serve as a keto side dish.

Enjoy!

Nutrition: calories 80, fat 1, fiber 2, carbs 1, protein 4

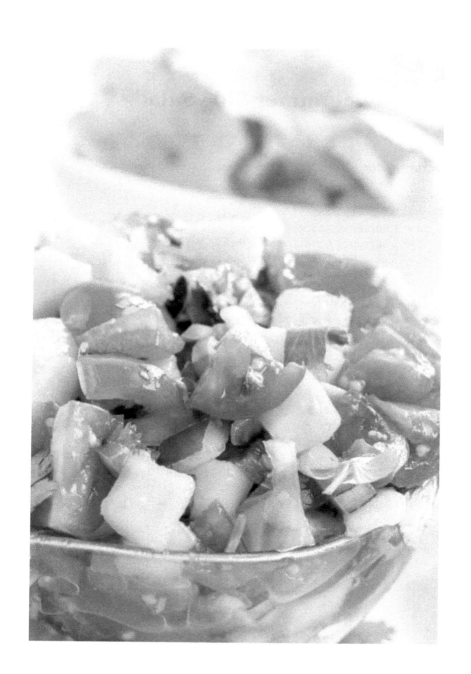

Summer Side Salad

It's going to be the best summer side salad ever!

Preparation time: 10 minutes **Cooking time:** 5 minutes **Servings:** 6

Ingredients:
- ½ cup extra virgin olive oil
- 1 cucumber, chopped
- 2 baguettes, cut into small cubes
- 2 pints colored cherry tomatoes, cut in halves
- Salt and black pepper to the taste
- 1 red onion, chopped
- 3 tablespoons balsamic vinegar
- 1 garlic clove, minced
- 1 bunch basil, roughly chopped

Directions:
1. In a bowl, mix bread cubes with half of the oil and toss to coat.
2. Heat up a pan over medium high heat, add bread, stir, toast for 10 minutes, take off heat, drain and leave aside for now.
3. In a bowl, mix vinegar with salt, pepper and the rest of the oil and whisk very well.
4. In a salad bowl mix cucumber with tomatoes, onion, garlic and bread.
5. Add vinegar dressing, toss to coat, sprinkle basil, add more salt and pepper if needed, toss to coat and serve.

Enjoy!

Nutrition: calories 90, fat 0, fiber 2, carbs 2, protein 4

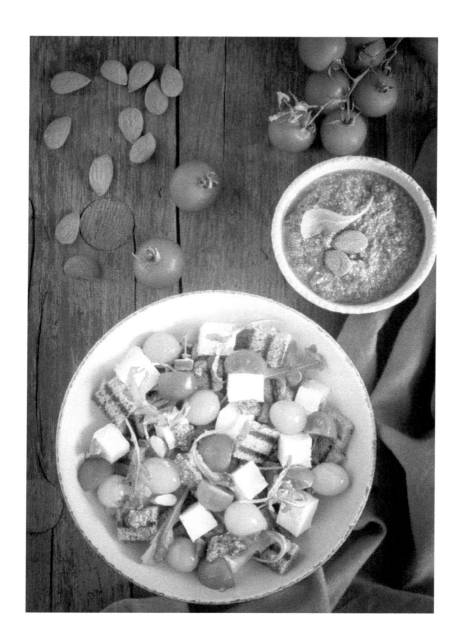

Tomato And Bocconcini

This salad goes really well with a grilled steak!

Preparation time: 6 minutes **Cooking time:** 0 minutes **Servings:** 4

Ingredients:
- 20 ounces tomatoes, cut in wedges
- 2 tablespoons extra virgin olive oil
- 1 and ½ tablespoons balsamic vinegar
- 1 teaspoon stevia
- 1 garlic clove, finely minced
- 8 ounces baby bocconcini, drain and torn
- 1 cup basil leaves, roughly chopped
- Salt and black pepper to the taste

Directions:
1. In a bowl, mix stevia with vinegar, garlic, oil, salt and pepper and whisk very well.
2. In a salad bowl, mix bocconcini with tomato and basil.
3. Add dressing, toss to coat and serve right away as a keto side dish.

Enjoy!

Nutrition: calories 100, fat 2, fiber 2, carbs 1, protein 9

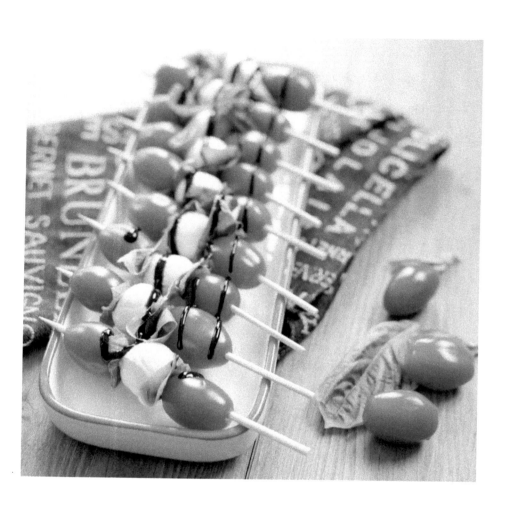

Cucumber And Dates Salad

This is a very healthy keto side salad! Try it and enjoy its taste!

Preparation time: 10 minutes **Cooking time:** 0 minutes **Servings:** 4

Ingredients:
- 2 English cucumbers, chopped
- 8 dates, pitted and sliced
- ¾ cup fennel, thinly sliced
- 2 tablespoons chives, finely chopped
- ½ cup walnuts, chopped
- 2 tablespoons lemon juice
- 4 tablespoons fruity olive oil
- Salt and black pepper to the taste

Directions:
1. Put cucumber pieces on a paper towel, press well and transfer to a salad bowl.
2. Crush them a bit using a fork.
3. Add dates, fennel, chives and walnuts and stir gently.
4. Add salt, pepper to the taste, lemon juice and the oil, toss to coat and serve right away.

Enjoy!

Nutrition: calories 80, fat 0.2, fiber 1, carbs 0.4, protein 5

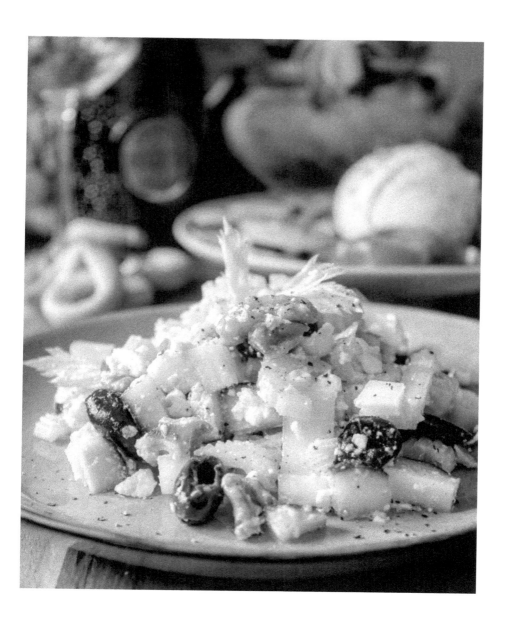

Easy Eggplant Salad

It's a good idea for a light keto side dish!

Preparation time: 10 minutes **Cooking time:** 10 minutes **Servings:** 4

Ingredients:
- 1 eggplant, sliced
- 1 red onion, sliced
- A drizzle of canola oil
- 1 avocado, pitted and chopped
- 1 teaspoon mustard
- 1 tablespoon balsamic vinegar
- 1 tablespoon fresh oregano, chopped
- A drizzle of olive oil
- Salt and black pepper to the taste
- Zest from 1 lemon
- Some parsley sprigs, chopped for serving

Directions:
1. Brush red onion slices and eggplant ones with a drizzle of canola oil, place them on heated kitchen grill and cook them until they become soft.
2. Transfer them to a cutting board, leave them to cool down, chop them and put them in a bowl.
3. Add avocado and stir gently.
4. In a bowl, mix vinegar with mustard, oregano, olive oil, salt and pepper to the taste.
5. Add this to eggplant, avocado and onion mix, toss to coat, add lemon zest and parsley on top and serve.

Enjoy!

Nutrition: calories 120, fat 3, fiber 2, carbs 1, protein 8

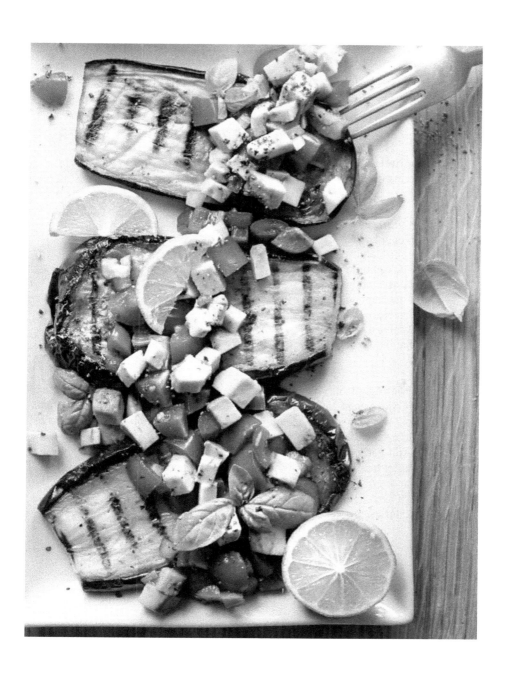

Special Side Salad

We really like this Italian style side salad!

Preparation time: 2 hours and 10 minutes **Cooking time:** 1 hour and 30 minutes **Servings:** 12

Ingredients:
- 1 garlic clove, crushed
- 6 eggplants
- 1 teaspoon parsley, dried
- 1 teaspoon oregano, dried
- ¼ teaspoon basil, dried
- 3 tablespoons extra virgin olive oil
- 2 tablespoons stevia
- 1 tablespoon balsamic vinegar
- Salt and black pepper to the taste

Directions:
1. Prick eggplants with a fork, arrange them on a baking sheet, introduce in the oven at 350 degrees F, bake for 1 hour and 30 minutes, take them out of the oven, leave them to cool down, peel, chop them and transfer to a salad bowl.
2. Add garlic, oil, parsley, stevia, oregano, basil, salt and pepper to the taste, toss to coat, keep in the fridge for 2 hours and then serve.

Enjoy!

Nutrition: calories 150, fat 1, fiber 2, carbs 1, protein 8

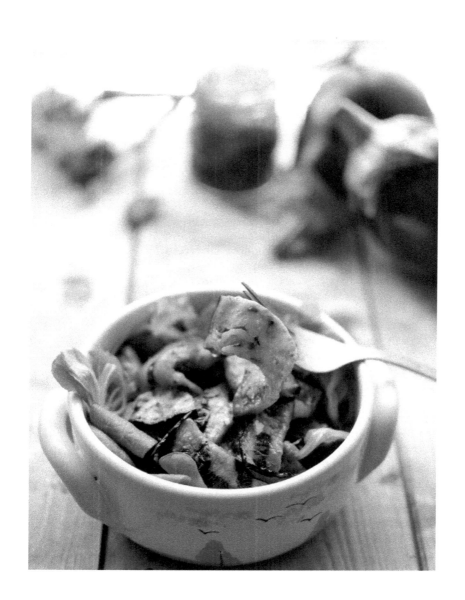

Special Endives And Watercress Side Salad

It's such a fresh side dish that goes with a keto grilled steak!

Preparation time: 10 minutes **Cooking time:** 5 minutes **Servings:** 4

Ingredients:
- 4 medium endives, roots and ends cut and thinly sliced crosswise
- 1 tablespoon lemon juice
- 1 shallot finely, chopped
- 1 tablespoon balsamic vinegar
- 2 tablespoons extra virgin olive oil
- 6 tablespoons heavy cream
- Salt and black pepper to the taste
- 4 ounces watercress, cut in medium springs
- 1 apple, thinly sliced
- 1 tablespoon chervil, chopped
- 1 tablespoon tarragon, chopped
- 1 tablespoon chives, chopped
- 1/3 cup almonds, chopped
- 1 tablespoon parsley, chopped

Directions:
1. In a bowl, mix lemon juice with vinegar, salt and shallot, stir and leave a side for 10 minutes.
2. Add olive oil, pepper, stir and leave aside for another 2 minutes.
3. Put endives, apple, watercress, chives, tarragon, parsley and chervil in a salad bowl.
4. Add salt and pepper to the taste and toss to coat.
5. Add heavy cream and vinaigrette, stir gently and serve as a side dish with almonds on top.

Enjoy!

Nutrition: calories 200, fat 3, fiber 5, carbs 2, protein 10

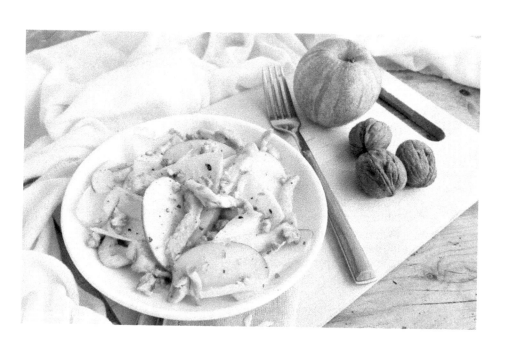

Indian Side Salad

It's very healthy and rich!

Preparation time: 15 minutes **Cooking time:** 0 minutes **Servings:** 6

Ingredients:
- 3 carrots, finely grated
- 2 courgettes, finely sliced
- A bunch of radishes, finely sliced
- ½ red onion, chopped
- 6 mint leaves, roughly chopped

For the salad dressing:
- 1 teaspoon mustard
- 1 tablespoons homemade mayo
- 1 tablespoons balsamic vinegar
- 2 tablespoons extra virgin olive oil
- Salt and black pepper to the taste

Directions:
1. In a bowl, mix mustard with mayo, vinegar, salt and pepper to the taste and stir well.
2. Add oil gradually and whisk everything.
3. In a salad bowl, mix carrots with radishes, courgettes and mint leaves.
4. Add salad dressing, toss to coat and keep in the fridge until you serve it.

Enjoy!

Nutrition: calories 140, fat 1, fiber 2, carbs 1, protein 7

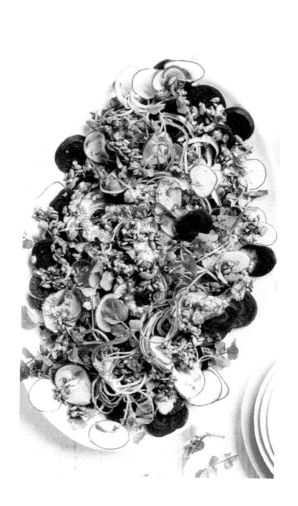

Conclusion

This is really a life changing cookbook. It shows you everything you need to know about the Ketogenic diet and it helps you get started.

You now know some of the best and most popular Ketogenic recipes in the world.

We have something for everyone's taste!

So, don't hesitate too much and start your new life as a follower of the Ketogenic diet!

Get your hands on this special recipes collection and start cooking in this new, exciting and healthy way!

Have a lot of fun and enjoy your Ketogenic diet!

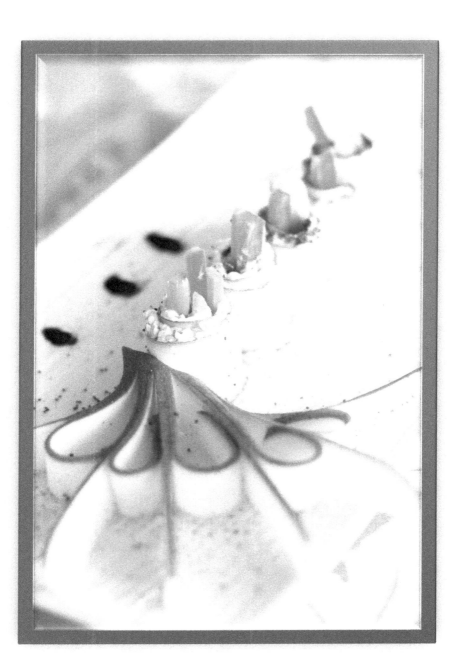